# Contents

# Introduction

Welcome to the world of cannabis-infused cooking! This cookbook is your ultimate guide to exploring the wonderful realm of culinary creations with cannabis as the star ingredient. Whether you're a seasoned cannabis connoisseur or someone curious about incorporating cannabis into your cooking repertoire, this ebook will provide you with a wealth of information, recipes, and tips to enhance your culinary adventures.

## About This Cookbook

In this section, we'll introduce you to the purpose and scope of this cookbook. You'll learn about the goals and objectives we have set for this book, as well as the intended audience. We aim to provide a comprehensive resource that educates, inspires, and empowers readers to confidently cook with cannabis.

## The Basics of Cooking with Cannabis

If you're new to cooking with cannabis, fear not! We'll cover all the basics to get you started. You'll learn about decarboxylation, the process of activating the cannabinoids in cannabis through heat, which is crucial for unlocking its therapeutic and psychoactive effects. We'll guide you through the various methods of infusing cannabis into oils, butters, and tinctures, and explain their different uses in cooking.

# Understanding Cannabis Strains and Types

Cannabis comes in a variety of strains, each with its own unique combination of cannabinoids and terpenes, which contribute to its flavor, aroma, and effects. In this section, we'll delve into the different types of cannabis strains, including indicas, sativas, and hybrids, and discuss how their characteristics can influence your culinary creations. You'll gain a deeper understanding of the plant and how to select the right strain for your desired outcome.

## Dosage and Potency Considerations

Cooking with cannabis requires careful consideration of dosage and potency to ensure a pleasant and controlled experience. We'll provide you with essential information on calculating and measuring the potency of your cannabis-infused dishes. Understanding the potency will help you adjust your recipes to achieve the desired effects without overwhelming your taste buds or compromising safety.

## Safety Precautions and Legal Considerations

As with any cooking endeavor, safety is paramount. We'll highlight important safety precautions you should follow when working with cannabis, including proper storage, handling, and labeling. Additionally, we'll touch on the legal landscape surrounding cannabis and provide general guidelines to help you navigate the laws and regulations specific to your jurisdiction.

# Cannabis Infused Oils, Butters, and Tinctures

Now that you're familiar with the basics, it's time to explore the various methods of infusing cannabis into oils, butters, and tinctures. These versatile cannabis-infused bases form the foundation for countless recipes and allow you to incorporate cannabis seamlessly into your culinary creations. In this section, we'll cover the following:

## Homemade Cannabis-Infused Oil

Learn how to make your own cannabis-infused oil at home using different extraction methods such as heat infusion, cold infusion, or using a cannabis-infused concentrate. We'll guide you through the step-by-step process, including selecting the right oil, decarboxylation, infusion techniques, and storage tips. You'll be equipped with the knowledge to create your own infused oils, perfect for sautéing, dressing, or drizzling over your favorite dishes.

## Cannabis-Infused Butter

Butter is a beloved ingredient in many culinary recipes, and infusing it with cannabis opens up a world of possibilities. We'll explore various methods of infusing butter with cannabis, including stovetop methods, slow cooker techniques, and using cannabis concentrates. You'll discover how to incorporate cannabis-infused butter into baked goods, pastries, sauces, and more, adding a delightful twist to your favorite recipes.

# Cannabis Tinctures and Extracts

Tinctures and extracts are concentrated forms of cannabis that offer precise dosing and versatile applications. In this section, we'll guide you through the process of making cannabis tinctures using alcohol or glycerin as solvents. You'll learn about the different extraction methods, dosage considerations, and creative ways to use cannabis tinctures in your beverages and recipes.

By mastering the art of cannabis-infused oils, butters, and tinctures, you'll have the foundation to embark on a culinary journey filled with exciting flavors and experiences. In the following sections, we'll dive into specific recipes for appetizers, main dishes, side dishes, desserts, beverages, and more, where you can put your cannabis-infused bases to use and unleash your creativity in the kitchen.

Stay tuned for the next sections, where we'll explore delicious recipes that showcase the versatility and potential of cooking with cannabis. Get ready to elevate your culinary skills and embark on a flavorful adventure like no other!

# Cannabis Cooking Tips and Tricks

Cooking with cannabis opens up a world of flavors, aromas, and experiences. To ensure your cannabis-infused dishes are a success, there are several important tips and tricks to keep in mind. In this section, we'll explore proper storage and labeling techniques, enhancing flavors with cannabis, and calculating and adjusting dosage for a controlled and enjoyable culinary adventure.

## Proper Storage and Labeling

Proper storage of cannabis-infused ingredients and finished dishes is essential to maintain freshness, potency, and safety. Here are some key tips for storing your cannabis and cannabis-infused products:

Store cannabis in a cool, dry, and dark place: Light, heat, and moisture can degrade the quality of cannabis and diminish its potency. Keep your cannabis in an airtight container away from direct sunlight or heat sources.

Label your cannabis-infused ingredients and products: Clearly label your cannabis-infused oils, butters, tinctures, and any prepared dishes with the strain used, date of preparation, and dosage per serving. This helps you keep track of potency and ensures safe consumption.

Keep cannabis-infused products out of reach of children and pets: Make sure to store your cannabis-infused ingredients and finished dishes in a secure location, away from the reach of children and pets. Consider using childproof containers for added safety.

Follow local regulations: Be aware of the legal requirements regarding cannabis storage and labeling in your jurisdiction. Different regions may have specific guidelines for packaging, dosage limits, and labeling information.

By implementing proper storage and labeling practices, you can maintain the quality and potency of your cannabis-infused ingredients, while also ensuring the safety of yourself and others.

## Enhancing Flavors with Cannabis

Cannabis possesses a range of flavors and aromas that can complement and enhance various dishes.

Here are some tips for incorporating cannabis flavors into your culinary creations:

Experiment with different strains: Different cannabis strains have unique flavor profiles, ranging from fruity and citrusy to earthy and herbal. Select strains that complement the flavors of your dish or experiment with contrasting flavors to create interesting combinations.

Infuse oils or butter with additional herbs and spices: When preparing cannabis-infused oils or butter, consider adding complementary herbs and spices to enhance the overall flavor. For example, infusing cannabis with rosemary, thyme, or garlic can add depth and complexity to savory dishes.

Use terpene-rich strains: Terpenes are aromatic compounds found in cannabis that contribute to its distinct flavors. Seek out strains that are high in terpenes such as limonene, myrcene, or pinene, which can add citrusy, fruity, or piney notes to your recipes.

Consider the extraction method: The extraction method you choose for your cannabis-infused ingredients can affect the flavor profile. For example, using a cold infusion method may result in a milder cannabis flavor compared to a heat infusion method. Experiment with different extraction techniques to find the flavor balance that suits your preferences.

Remember, when infusing cannabis into your dishes, start with a small amount and gradually increase to achieve the desired flavor intensity. It's important to strike a balance between the cannabis flavor and the overall taste of your recipe.

## Calculating and Adjusting Dosage

Accurately calculating and adjusting the dosage of your cannabis-infused dishes is crucial for a safe and enjoyable experience. Here are some tips to help you determine and modify the potency of your recipes:

Understand the potency of your cannabis: Knowing the potency of your cannabis is essential for accurate dosage calculations. If you're using store-bought cannabis, check the label for the THC and CBD percentages. If you're unsure, consider getting your cannabis tested at a reputable lab for precise potency information.

Start low and go slow: When cooking with cannabis, it's advisable to start with a low dosage, especially if you're new to cannabis-infused edibles. Begin with small portions or servings to gauge your tolerance and the effects. Remember that the onset and duration of effects can vary, so be patient and give the cannabis-infused dish time to take effect before consuming more.

Adjust recipes based on desired potency: If you want to increase or decrease the potency of a recipe, you can adjust the amount of cannabis-infused ingredient used. For example, if a recipe calls for one tablespoon of cannabis-infused oil, you can reduce it to half a tablespoon for a milder potency or increase it to one and a half tablespoons for a stronger effect. Keep in mind that the potency may vary based on factors such as strain, decarboxylation, and infusion method.

Keep track of dosage per serving: To ensure consistent dosing, calculate the dosage per serving in your recipes. Divide the total amount of cannabis used by the number of servings to determine the approximate dosage per portion. This information is crucial for labeling your dishes and communicating the potency to others.

Remember, the effects of cannabis-infused edibles can be more potent and long-lasting compared to other consumption methods. Always exercise caution, start with low dosages, and be aware of your personal tolerance and sensitivity to cannabis.

By following these cannabis cooking tips and tricks, you'll be well-equipped to create delicious and potent cannabis-infused dishes. Enjoy your culinary explorations responsibly, and remember to respect the legal regulations and guidelines in your area.

# Cannabis Infused Gummies

This recipe for cannabis infused gummies makes a large amount of gummies. This is great for microdosing or if you like to eat a lot of gummies. The secret to making this successfully is to whisk lots and keep it boiling.

Course: Snack

Cuisine: Canadian

Keyword: gummy


Prep Time: 10 minutes

Cook Time: 10 minutes

Total Time: 20 minutes

Servings: 72 Gummies

Calories: 9kcal

Ingredients

- 1 pack Flavored Jello 3 ounce

- 1 dram Extra Flavor (if desired)

- 28 g Gelatin

- 2 tsp Soy Lecithin

- 8 tbsp Infused Coconut Oil

- 1 3/4 cup Water, divided

Instructions

1. Combine Cannabis Infused Coconut Oil, Soy Lecithin and 3/4 cup of water in a saucepan. Heat on low-medium until all blended.

2. Add gelatin to 1 cup of boiling water, whisk thoroughly.

3. Add Jello package to gelatin water and whisk thoroughly.

4. Add the gelatin/water/jello mix to the pot with the oil/lecithin/water and bring to a boil over medium heat, whisking briskly. Continue whisking boiling mixture for 6 minutes, adjusting heat as needed to prevent over/under boiling.

5. Remove from heat and let mixture cool slightly before pouring into molds.

6. Allow 2 hours to completely cool at room temperature.

7. Remove gummy candies from molds and allow to air dry for 48 to 60 hours. Turn gummy candies over if tops are shrinking faster than the rest of the gummy.

Notes

Dosage

Consume 1 Gummy candy every 2 to 4 hours.

Nutrition

Serving: 2.6g | Calories: 9kcal

# Cannabis Tapioca Pudding Recipe

Cannabis tapioca pudding is easy to make, especially if you have cannamilk in your fridge. Ingredients are simple and include Minit Tapioca, cannamilk, egg, sugar and vanilla.

0 from 0 votes

Course: Dessert

Cuisine: South American

Keyword: cannabis infused, pudding, tapioca

Prep Time: 5 minutes

Cook Time: 5 minutes

Servings: 4

Calories: 185kcal

## Equipment

- Saucepan

## Ingredients

- 2 3/4 c cannamilk

- 1/4 c sugar

- 3 Tbsp Minit Tapioca

- 1 egg, slightly beaten

- 1 tsp vanilla extract

## Instructions

1. Add cannamilk, sugar, tapioca and egg to a medium saucepan. Stir together and let sit for 5 minutes.

2. Bring mixture to a full boil while stirring constantly. Remove from heat. Stir in vanilla. Cool for 20 minutes without stirring.

3. Serve warm or chilled.

Notes

Microwave Instructions

Put cannamilk, sugar, egg, and minit tapioca into a large microwavable bowl. Let mixture sit for 5 minutes. Microwave 10 to 12 minutes on high, stirring every 3 minutes, until mixture comes to a boil. Add vanilla. Do not stir for 20 minutes. Cool to desired temperature.

Nutrition

Calories: 185kcal

# Wake and Bake Cannabis Pancakes Recipe

Wake and Bake Cannabis Pancakes can be made with cannamilk, yogurt whey, cannabutter or tincture. The fluffy, soft pancakes are delicious with any toppings. Enjoy them as meals, snacks or desserts.

0 from 0 votes

Course: Breakfast

Cuisine: American, Canadian, Dutch

Keyword: cannamilk, cannapancakes, pancakes

Prep Time: 5 minutes

Cook Time: 10 minutes

Servings: 10 pancakes

Calories: 140kcal

## Equipment

- Non-stick frying pan

- Mixing Bowls

- Wooden Spoon

## Ingredients

- 1 1/3 c all-purpose flour

- 3 Tbsp sugar

- 2 1/2 tsp baking powder

- 1/2 tsp salt

- 1 1/4 c cannamilk

- 1 large egg, slightly beaten

- 3 Tbsp melted butter or oil

- 1/4 tsp vanilla extract

- additional oil for frying

Instructions

1. In a mixing bowl, combine flour, sugar, baking powder and salt. Make a well in the center of the bowl.

2. In another mixing bowl combine slightly beaten egg, cannamilk (or whey), oil (or melted butter) and vanilla. Add ingredients to the well in the bowl of dry ingredients.

3. Mix together only until incorporated and batter is slightly lumpy. Over-mixing causes flat and chewy cannabis pancakes due to the development of gluten.

4. Using 1/3 cup batter for each cannabis pancake, pour into greased and preheated non-stick pan on medium heat. When bubbles form and pop, check to see that the pancake is nicely browned, then flip. When the other side is nicely browned, remove pancakes from pan.

5. Add more oil to the pan. Continue cooking with a generous amount of oil until all pancakes are done.

6. Serve immediately or cool and store in the fridge or freezer for later use.

7. Always indicate that this food contains THC and keep out of reach of children and pets.

Notes

Variations of Easy Infused Cannabis Pancakes

1. You can make Wake and Bake Cannabis Pancakes with regular milk or whey , then add infused toppings.

2. You can substitute cannabis tincture in place of an equal amount of oil/melted butter in the recipe.

Nutrition

Calories: 140kcal

# Super Easy Cannabis Chocolate Recipe

If you don't have a lot of time to spend in the kitchen, super easy cannabis chocolate is not complicated and contains only a few ingredients.

4.59 from 89 votes

Course: Dessert

Cuisine: American, Canadian

Keyword: cannabis chocolate, chocolate

Prep Time: 5 minutes

Cook Time: 15 minutes

Servings: 12

Calories: 134kcal

Author: Dee Rina

Equipment

- Chocolate Molds

- Double Boiler

Ingredients

- 300 g chocolate chips or baking chocolate

- decarboxylated cannabis or activated tincture use preferred dose

## Instructions

1. Heat baking chocolate or chocolate chips in a bowl placed on top of a pot of hot water. The bowl must have a larger diameter than the pot to prevent water from contaminating the chocolate. Do not cover the bowl when heating chocolate.

2. Once the chocolate melts and has a runny consistency, add the ground decarbed cannabis or activated tincture. Mix very well. Continue to heat gently until you have a smooth pourable consistency.

3. Pour into chocolate molds being careful not to get any water in the chocolate. Let chocolates cool at room temperature.

## Notes

### Lecithin

You can add lecithin granules to increase the viscosity of chocolate, making it easier to pour.

### Do Not Add Liquids

Do not add honey, syrup, vanilla extract or any other liquids to chocolate.

### Nutrition

Calories: 134kcal

## Creamy Cannabis Rice Pudding

Made with cannamilk, creamy cannabis rice pudding is naturally gluten-free. It can be eaten as either a meal or a dessert. Plus, it and tastes great hot or cold.

0 from 0 votes

Course: Dessert

Cuisine: American, Canadian

Keyword: canna rice pudding, gluten-free, rice pudding

Prep Time: 5 minutes

Cook Time: 40 minutes

Total Time: 45 minutes

Servings: 4

Calories: 305kcal

Author: Dee Rina

Ingredients

- 3/4 c uncooked rice

- 2 c cannamilk, divided

- 1/3 c granulated white sugar

- 1/4 tsp salt

- 1 egg

- 2/3 c golden raisins

- 1/2 tsp cinnamon

- 1/8 tsp cloves

- 1/8 tsp nutmeg

- 1/2 tsp vanilla extract

- 1 Tbsp butter

## Instructions

1. Bring 1 ½ cups water and uncooked rice to a boil. Simmer for 20 minutes.

2. While rice is cooking, heat 1 1/2 cups cannamilk, sugar and salt in a saucepan on low until rice is done.

3. Add rice to the heated mixture and cook on medium until it becomes thick and creamy.

4. Whisk together the remaining 1/2 cup cannamilk, egg, cinnamon, cloves and nutmeg. Add to thickened mixture along with raisins, if using. Boil on medium heat for 3 minutes, stirring constantly.

5. Remove from heat. Stir in butter and vanilla. Let cool. Serve warm or cold

Notes

## Vegan Friendly Creamy Cannabis Rice Pudding

Use coconut cannamilk, vegan margarine and cornstarch to thicken, eliminating the dairy and egg of the original recipe. If the coconut cannamilk is very thick, leave out the cornstarch also.

## Egg-Free Creamy Canna Rice Pudding

Use cornstarch instead of the egg to thicken. Whisk 1/2 Tbsp cornstarch into the second addition of cannamilk.

Nutrition

Serving: 0g | Calories: 305kcal | Carbohydrates: 0g | Protein: 0g | Fat: 0g | Saturated Fat: 0g | Polyunsaturated Fat: 0g | Monounsaturated Fat: 0g | Trans Fat: 0g | Cholesterol: 0mg | Sodium: 0mg | Potassium: 0mg | Fiber: 0g | Sugar: 0g | Vitamin A: 0IU | Vitamin C: 0mg | Calcium: 0mg | Iron: 0mg

## Easy Cannabis Chocolate Fudge

This is an easy cannabis chocolate fudge recipe that takes only 10 minutes to prepare. Use either the small batch or the regular batch for delicious, sweet, gluten-free edibles.

4.75 from 35 votes

Course: Dessert

Cuisine: American

Keyword: chocolate, fudge

Prep Time: 5 minutes

Cook Time: 5 minutes

Total Time: 10 minutes

Servings: 24

Calories: 182kcal

Author: Dee Rina

Ingredients

# Regular Batch Cannabis Chocolate Fudge

## Ingredients

- 3 c Semisweet chocolate chips
- 14 oz Sweetened condensed milk
- 1/4 c Cannabutter

## Instructions

Regular Batch Cannabis Chocolate Fudge Instructions

1. Spray 8" x 8" baking pan lightly with cooking oil.

2. Put all ingredients into a microwave safe mixing bowl. Cook on high for 5 minutes, stopping to stir once or twice. Stir well. Pour into prepared pan. Cool. Cut into 24 equal sized pieces.

## Notes

## Small Batch Cannabis Chocolate Fudge Ingredients

- 1 1/2 cups Semisweet chocolate chips

- 7 ounces Sweetened condensed milk

- 2 Tbsp Cannabutter

## Small Batch Cannabis Chocolate Fudge Instructions

- Prepare loaf pan by lining with foil or parchment and spray lightly with cooking spray.

- Put all ingredients into microwave safe mixing bowl. Heat on high for 1 1/2 to 2 minutes. Stir. Heat on high for another 2 minutes. Stir well. Pour into prepared pan. Cool. Lift from pan. Cut into 12 equal sized pieces.

# Flavor Variation - Cannabis Mint Chocolate Fudge

Add a few drops of LorAnn mint oil before heating to make mint chocolate fudge.

Nutrition

Serving: 0g | Calories: 182kcal | Carbohydrates: 0g | Protein: 0g | Fat: 0g | Saturated Fat: 0g | Polyunsaturated Fat: 0g | Monounsaturated Fat: 0g | Trans Fat: 0g | Cholesterol: 0mg | Sodium: 0mg | Potassium: 0mg | Fiber: 0g | Sugar: 0g | Vitamin A: 0IU | Vitamin C: 0mg | Calcium: 0mg | Iron: 0mg

# Cannabis Peanut Butter Cookies

## Gluten-Free

Gluten-free cannabis peanut butter cookies have only 4 simple ingredients. These flourless cookies are easy to make whether you are on a gluten-free diet or not.

4.8 from 5 votes

Course: Dessert

Cuisine: American

Keyword: cannabis peanut butter cookies

Prep Time: 5 minutes

Cook Time: 20 minutes

Total Time: 25 minutes

Servings: 18 cookies

Calories: 130kcal

Author: Dee Rina

## Ingredients

- 1 cup cannabis peanut butter

- 1 cup granulated sugar

- 1 egg

- 1 tsp vanilla

## Instructions

1. Preheat oven to 350°F.

2. Mix all ingredients together in a mixing bowl.

3. Divide into 18 equal portions. Roll into balls. Space out evenly on 2 parchment-lined cookie sheets. Press dough with a fork to create lines. Sprinkle with sugar if desired.

4. Bake each sheet separately in the oven for 10 minutes.

5. Cool on cookie sheet for 5 minutes, then remove to cooling rack until completely cooled.

Notes

How To Make Infused Peanut Butter

If you don't have infused peanut butter, you can easily make some by mixing tincture, decarbed dried flower or decarbed concentrates dissolved in oil with peanut butter. Use a wooden spoon or hand mixer to thoroughly mix cannabis into peanut butter.

## Nutrition

Serving: 0g | Calories: 130kcal | Carbohydrates: 0g | Protein: 0g | Fat: 0g | Saturated Fat: 0g | Polyunsaturated Fat: 0g | Monounsaturated Fat: 0g | Trans Fat: 0g | Cholesterol: 0mg | Sodium: 0mg | Potassium: 0mg | Fiber: 0g | Sugar: 0g | Vitamin A: 0IU | Vitamin C: 0mg | Calcium: 0mg | Iron: 0mg

# Cannabis Sticky Buns

Cannabis sticky buns can be made easily with simple ingredients. The dough is not complicated and goes together easily. If you love your buns sticky, there is no shortage of ooey gooey goodness here.

5 from 3 votes

Course: Dessert

Cuisine: Danish, Swedish

Keyword: cannabis sticky buns, sticky buns

Prep Time: 2 hours 30 minutes

Cook Time: 45 minutes

Rising: 2 hours 30 minutes

Total Time: 3 hours 15 minutes

Servings: 12

Calories: 431kcal

Author: Joe Balazs

Ingredients

Dough Ingredients

- 1 1/4 cup Milk or Cannamilk at 105°F

- 2 1/4 tsp Instant Dry Yeast

- 1/4 cup Granulated Sugar

- 1 Large Egg, Room Temperature

- 1/4 cup Unsalted Butter or Cannabutter, melted

- 3 1/2 cup all-purpose flour

- 3/4 tsp Salt

Goo Ingredients

- 1/2 cup Unsalted Butter or Cannabutter

- 1 cup Brown Sugar

- 1/2 cup Maple Syrup

Filling Ingredients

- 1 cup Brown Sugar

- 1 1/2 Tbsp Ground Cinnamon

- 1/4 cup Butter or Cannabutter

Instructions

Dough Making Instructions

1. Measure all ingredients into a mixing bowl.

2. Mix with stand mixer and dough hook until combined, then knead for 3 minutes.

By hand, mix with a wooden spoon and knead for 5 minutes.

3. Place dough into greased bowl, cover with plastic wrap and let rise for 1 1/2 to 2 hours.

Goo Making Instructions

1. Mix all ingredients together and spread evenly in the bottom of 9" x 13" pan. Set aside.

Making The Filling

1. Mix all filling ingredients together. Set Aside.

Assembling Canna Sticky Buns

1. Roll risen dough out into a 12" x 18" rectangle.

2. Spread filling evenly over dough rectangle.

3. Roll up dough starting on the long side

4. Cut roll into 12 equal sized pieces and space out evenly on top of the goo in the 9" x 13" pan.

5. Cover with a towel and let rolls rise for 1 hour.

Baking Sticky Buns

1. Preheat oven to 350°F.

2. Remove towel from risen sticky buns. Put in preheated oven and bake for 40 to 45 minutes.

3. Remove from oven and place pan on cooling rack for 15 minutes

4. Invert onto large serving plate.

5. Enjoy in moderation.

Notes

# Wake and Bake Cannabis Sticky Buns

After cutting roll into 12 pieces and placing in the pan on top of the goo, cover pan and put in the fridge overnight. In the morning, place pan into a cold oven. Preheat oven to 350°F and continue baking for 40 to 45 minutes. Remove from oven and set on a cooling rack for 15 minutes. Invert and serve.

Nutrition

Serving: 0g | Calories: 431kcal | Carbohydrates: 0g | Protein: 0g | Fat: 0g | Saturated Fat: 0g | Polyunsaturated Fat: 0g | Monounsaturated Fat: 0g | Trans Fat: 0g | Cholesterol: 0mg | Sodium: 0mg | Potassium: 0mg | Fiber: 0g | Sugar: 0g | Vitamin A: 0IU | Vitamin C: 0mg | Calcium: 0mg | Iron: 0mg

# Cannahoney Recipe

The main thing that sets this cannahoney recipe apart from other cannahoney recipes is the use of sunflower lecithin. Also, there is no cheesecloth required, there is less mess, less time and less energy required to make this infused cannahoney.

4.72 from 7 votes

Course: Dessert

Cuisine: Canadian

Keyword: cannahoney

Prep Time: 10 minutes

Total Time: 10 minutes

Servings: 16 Tablespoons

Calories: 75kcal

Ingredients

- 1 cup creamed honey

- 1 Tbsp liquid coconut oil

- 1 Tbsp sunflower lecithin

- cannabis

- LorAnn flavored oil optional

Instructions

1. Decarboxylate dried cannabis flower or concentrates. Grind cannabis to a fine powder. If

using concentrates, dissolve in 1 Tbsp warm coconut oil.

2. Mix coconut oil, sunflower lecithin, cannabis and flavoring until it is smooth and there are no lumps.

3. Add honey to oil/lecithin/cannabis mixture. Cream together until mixture is smooth and completely incorporated.

4. Put cannahoney in jar. Store in a cool, dark place.

Notes

Using Dried Cannabis Flower to Make Cannahoney

Grind decarboxylated cannabis flower to a fine powder. Add to lecithin, coconut oil and flavoring.

Using Capsules or Tincture to Make Cannahoney

Put tincture or capsules into a tablespoon and top up with liquid coconut oil totaling 1 Tbsp oil.

## Using Concentrates to Make Cannahoney

You can use BHO, shatter, RSO and other concentrates to make cannahoney. After decarboxylation, dissolve concentrates in one Tbsp of warm liquid coconut oil. Do not add additional coconut oil to the cannahoney.

## Nutrition

Serving: 0g | Calories: 75kcal | Carbohydrates: 0g | Protein: 0g | Fat: 0g | Saturated Fat: 0g | Polyunsaturated Fat: 0g | Monounsaturated Fat: 0g | Trans Fat: 0g | Cholesterol: 0mg | Sodium: 0mg | Potassium: 0mg | Fiber: 0g | Sugar: 0g | Vitamin A: 0IU | Vitamin C: 0mg | Calcium: 0mg | Iron: 0mg

# Cannabis Chocolate Pudding

This is a quick and easy recipe to make, especially if you have cannamilk on hand. Mix together dry ingredients in saucepan, slowly add cannamilk, boil, remove from heat, add remaining ingredients, divide into 4 equal portions, serve warm or cool and serve.

Cuisine: Canadian

Keyword: cannabis chocolate pudding

Prep Time: 5 minutes

Cook Time: 5 minutes

Total Time: 10 minutes

Servings: 4

Calories: 282kcal

Ingredients

- 2/3 cup sugar

- 1/4 cup cocoa powder

- 3 Tbsp cornstarch

- 1/4 tsp salt

- 2 1/4 cups cannamilk

- 2 Tbsp butter or margarine

- 1 tsp vanilla

- Whipped Topping optional

## Instructions

1. Stir sugar, cocoa, cornstarch and salt together in a medium saucepan over medium heat.

2. Slowly add cannamilk to dry ingredients in the saucepan. Use whisk if it becomes too lumpy.

3. Cook on medium heat and stir constantly until the mixture boils. Keep stirring and boil for one minute.

4. Remove from heat. Stir in butter and vanilla until well incorporated.

5. Pour equal portions of pudding into 4 small dishes or ramekins. Press plastic wrap onto pudding to prevent skin from forming on top. Serve warm or refrigerate for about 2 hours. Garnish with whipped topping, if desired.

## Notes

### Microwave Directions

In a large microwave safe bowl, combine sugar, cocoa, cornstarch and salt. Slowly mix in cannamilk. Microwave on high for 7 to 10 minutes until mixture boils. Be sure to stir every 2 minutes. Carefully remove from microwave. Stir in vanilla and butter. Pour into 4 serving dishes. Cool/refrigerate or eat warm.

### Variations

Instant Cannabis Chocolate Pudding

Mix cannamilk with instant pudding mix following package instructions.

Stovetop Cannabis Chocolate Pudding Mix

Mix cannamilk with stovetop pudding mix following package instructions.

Nutrition

Serving: 0g | Calories: 282kcal | Carbohydrates: 0g | Protein: 0g | Fat: 0g | Saturated Fat: 0g | Polyunsaturated Fat: 0g | Monounsaturated Fat: 0g | Trans Fat: 0g | Cholesterol: 0mg | Sodium: 0mg | Potassium: 0mg | Fiber: 0g | Sugar: 0g | Vitamin A: 0IU | Vitamin C: 0mg | Calcium: 0mg | Iron: 0mg

# Hungarian Crepes - Palacsinta

Cannabis infused Hungarian crepes or Palacsinta are a thin, delicate crepe with a creamy, sweet cottage cheese filling and topped with chocolate sauce. Serve as a dessert or as a meal.

4.5 from 2 votes

Course: Dessert, Main Course

Cuisine: Hungarian

Keyword: crepes, Hungarian crepes

Prep Time: 1 hour

Cook Time: 10 minutes

Total Time: 1 hour 10 minutes

Servings: 6

Calories: 418kcal

Author: Joe Balazs

Ingredients

Crepe Batter

- 3 Large eggs beaten

- 1 1/4 cups Cannamilk

- 3 Tbsp Melted Butter

- 1/4 tsp Salt

- 1 cup All-purpose flour

Filling

- 2 cups Cottage cheese

- 1/4 cup Icing sugar

- 1 Tbsp Lemon zest

- 1/2 tsp Vanilla extract

Chocolate Sauce

- 1 1/2 cups water

- 1 1/2 cups white sugar

- 1 cup Cocoa

- 1 dash Salt

- 1 tsp Vanilla extract

Instructions

Crepes

1. Using a medium mixing bowl, whisk together eggs, cannamilk, butter and salt. Whisk flour in, using small amounts at a time until well mixed and there are no lumps.

2. Refrigerate, covered for at least one hour. Make filling and topping while your batter is chilling.

3. Spread 1 tsp oil evenly over non-stick frying pan, using a paper towel to distribute evenly. Heat over medium heat.

4. Pour 1/4 cup of batter in center of pan and spread quickly by tilting and turning until the entire pan is evenly coated with a thin layer of batter.

5. When the batter starts to look dry after about 20 to 30 seconds, flip crepe over with a thin

spatula. Heat until slightly brown, about 10 to 15 seconds. Remove from pan.

6. Stack crepes on a plate, they will not stick together.

7. After all crepes are done, you can prepare them for serving. Place crepe on a flat surface, spread filling to within an inch of the edge and roll up. Drizzle with chocolate sauce.

Crepe Filling

1. Mix cottage cheese, icing sugar, lemon zest and vanilla in a bowl. Cover and refrigerate until needed.

Chocolate Sauce

1. Put water, white sugar, cocoa powder and salt in a saucepan. Heat over low heat while whisking

constantly until mixture simmers and thickens. Remove from heat and stir in vanilla. Serve warm or cold.

## Notes

### Savory Variation

Fill crepes with seasoned meat and top with gravy or sour cream.

## Nutrition

Serving: 0g | Calories: 418kcal | Carbohydrates: 0g | Protein: 0g | Fat: 0g | Saturated Fat: 0g | Polyunsaturated Fat: 0g | Monounsaturated Fat: 0g | Trans Fat: 0g | Cholesterol: 0mg | Sodium: 0mg | Potassium: 0mg | Fiber: 0g | Sugar: 0g |

Vitamin A: 0IU | Vitamin C: 0mg | Calcium: 0mg | Iron: 0mg

# Liquor Soaked Infused Cherries

Cannabis infused liquor soaked sour cherries are a luxurious treat for those who like to indulge on special occasions. The tartness, sweetness and smoothness are a refreshing jolt to the taste buds.

5 from 1 vote

Course: Dessert

Cuisine: Hungarian

Keyword: Infused Cherries, Liquor Soaked Infused Cherries

Prep Time: 30 minutes

Cook Time: 25 minutes

Infusion: 21 days

Total Time: 55 minutes

Servings: 4 servings

Calories: 0.218kcal

Author: Joe Balazs

Ingredients

- 2 cups sour cherries pitted

- 3 tbsp white sugar

- 4 tbsp infused liquor tincture

Instructions

1. Wash a 500 mL mason jar and sterilize by putting in the oven at 225° F for 20 minutes. Remove from oven and let cool. Remember not to touch the jar, it is very hot and will burn your skin. Sterilize lid by soaking in hot but not boiling water while you prepare the cherries.

2. Rinse cherries under cold water. Remove all stems and pits from the cherries.

3. Add about 1/3 of the cherries to the jar. Pour one Tablespoon of sugar over the cherries. Add the next 1/3 of cherries to the jar and pour one more tablespoon of sugar over. Add the last 1/3 of the cherries to the jar, leaving one inch headspace. Pour one Tablespoon of sugar over the cherries.

4. Pour 3 to 4 ounces of cannabis tincture over the cherries. If your tincture contains several doses of THC, then you can use a portion containing tincture and the remaining portion is straight alcohol. Seal jar tightly and shake gently to distribute the sugar and tincture throughout the cherries.

5. Store the container in the cupboard or pantry out of direct light for about 3 to 4 weeks to fully infuse. Gently shake the cherries once a week to distribute the sugar and liquid.

6. Refrigerate after opening. Store in fridge for several months, making sure that no children have access to the fridge.

7. Consume in moderation because cannabis can intensify the effects of alcohol.

8. Always label container to indicate that the contents contain THC.

Notes

Variation

You can use cherries with the pits inside, but you must poke a couple of pin holes in each cherry.

Nutrition

Serving: 0g | Calories: 0.218kcal | Carbohydrates: 0g | Protein: 0g | Fat: 0g | Saturated Fat: 0g | Polyunsaturated Fat: 0g | Monounsaturated Fat: 0g | Trans Fat: 0g | Cholesterol: 0mg | Sodium: 0mg | Potassium: 0mg | Fiber: 0g | Sugar: 0g | Vitamin A: 0IU | Vitamin C: 0mg | Calcium: 0mg | Iron: 0mg